CANCER AT A GLANCE

Essentials of Cancer Simplified

By

Jamie N. Luke

TABLE OF CONTENTS

INTRODUCTION

The human body is made up of cells, which are the fundamental structural components. Cells can grow and divide to produce new cells as the body requires them. In most cases, cells die or get damaged as they reach a certain point, when this happens; new cells emerge to take their place. Cancer develops when there is a disruption in the normally ordered progression of cell division, which leads to an unchecked increase in the number of cells. These cells have the potential to aggregate into a bulk known as a tumor. Two types of tumor exist: malignant and benign. Malignant tumors are those that have the potential to grow larger and metastasize, or spread to other areas of the body, while; benign tumors are those that grow but cannot spread.

The progression of some forms of cancer results in accelerated cell proliferation, whereas other types of cancer cause cells to proliferate and divide at a more gradual pace. While some types of cancer, like leukemia, do not result in the development of visible growths termed tumors, other types of cancer do. The vast majority of cells in the body are specialized and have predetermined lifespans. A phenomenon known as apoptosis is both normal and advantageous, although the death of cells may have the appearance of a negative impact. A cell receives a signal to die so that it can be replaced with a newer cell in the body that will perform its functions more effectively.

Cancerous cells lack the elements that notify them to cease dividing and to die when they reach a certain point, hence; they accumulate throughout the body, consuming the oxygen and nutrients that would normally be used by the body to sustain other cells. Cells that are cancerous have the potential to create tumors, weaken the immune system, and produce other alterations that interfere with the body's ability to perform its normal functions. It is possible for cancerous cells to begin in one location, then spread to other areas via the lymph nodes. These are groups of immune cells that can be found in many parts of the body.

An estimated 9.6 million deaths, or one in every six deaths, were attributed to cancer in 2018, making it the second highest cause of death worldwide. Men are more likely to develop lung, prostate, colorectal, stomach, and liver cancer than women, who are more likely to develop breast, colorectal, lung, cervical, and thyroid cancer.

The global burden of cancer continues to increase, putting an incredible amount of stress, both physically and emotionally, as well as financial pressure, on individuals, families, communities, and healthcare systems. A significant portion of the world's cancer patients do not have access to excellent diagnosis and treatment on time, and many of the world's health systems, particularly those in low- and middle-income nations, are the least prepared to deal with this burden.

The survival rates of many different types of cancer are improving in nations that have robust health systems. This is due to the increased availability of early diagnosis services, high-quality treatment options, and survivorship care.

CHAPTER I

Brief History of Cancer, What Is Cancer All About, Types of Cancer, How Cancer Spread, Where Cancer Can Spread To, Cancer Stages

BRIEF HISTORY OF CANCER

Cancer has been present in humans and other animals throughout recorded history, thus; it is not surprising that people have written about cancer since the dawn of history. Some of the earliest evidence of cancer has been discovered in fossilized bone tumors, ancient Egyptian human mummies, and ancient manuscripts. Mummies have been found to contain growths suggestive of osteosarcoma, a type of bone cancer. Bony skull destruction, as seen in head and neck cancer, has also been observed.

The origin of the word cancer is attributed to Hippocrates (460-370 BC), the "Father of Medicine" and Greek physician. Hippocrates referred to non-ulcer forming and ulcer forming tumors using the terms carcinos and carcinoma. In Greek, these words refer to a crab; they were most likely applied to the disease because cancer's finger-like projections evoked the shape of a crab. Celsus (25 BC - 50 AD), a Roman physician, later translated the Greek term into cancer, the Latin word for crab. Galen (130-200 AD), another Greek physician, utilized the Greek term oncos to describe tumors.

Although Hippocrates and Celsus continue to use the crab analogy to describe malignant tumors, Galen's term "oncos" is now part of the name for cancer specialists – oncologists.

Beginning in the 15th century, scientists gained a deeper understanding of the human body during the Renaissance. Galileo and Newton were among the first to employ the scientific method, which was later applied to the study of disease. Harvey's (1628) autopsies led to a previously unfathomable understanding of the circulation of blood through the heart and body. In 1761, Giovanni Morgagni of Padua was the first person to conduct autopsies in order to correlate a patient's illness with postmortem pathologic findings. This laid the groundwork for oncology, the scientific study of cancer.

Utilizing the modern microscope to study diseased tissues, the nineteenth century saw the birth of scientific oncology. Rudolf Virchow often referred to as the founder of cellular pathology, laid the scientific groundwork for the contemporary pathologic study of cancer. As Morgagni had correlated gross autopsy findings with the clinical course of diseases, so did Virchow correlate microscopic pathology with diseases. This technique not only facilitated a greater comprehension of the damage caused by cancer but also contributed to the development of cancer surgery. Now that the surgeon has removed body tissues for examination, a precise diagnosis can be made.

The pathologist could also inform the surgeon as to whether or not the cancer had been completely removed.

Oncology, the study of cancer, is the result of the efforts of countless scientists, physicians, and researchers from around the globe whose findings in anatomy, physiology, chemistry, epidemiology, and other related fields have shaped oncology into what it has become today. This field is one of the most rapidly evolving in modern medicine due to technological advancements and an ever-expanding understanding of cancer. The expansion of our understanding of the biology of cancer has led to remarkable advances in cancer early identification, treatment, and prevention. In the last two decades, scientists have learned more about cancer than in all the centuries preceding. This does not change the fact that all scientific knowledge is based on the hard work and discoveries of our predecessors, and we know there is still a great deal more to learn about cancer.

WHAT IS CANCER ALL ABOUT?

The following information will help you better comprehend what cancer is.

Humans are composed of trillions of cells that grow and divide as needed over the course of a lifetime. When cells become abnormal or age, they typically die. Cancer begins when this process goes awry and your cells continue to produce new cells while the old or abnormal ones do not die when they should.

As cancer cells multiply uncontrollably, they can crowd out healthy cells. This makes it difficult for your body to function normally. Cancer is a general term, ***"it describes the disease that can begin in almost any organ, tissue, or region of the body when abnormal cells grow uncontrollably, invade adjoining parts of the body and/or spread to other areas, and can infiltrate and destroy normal body tissue"***.

Cancer can develop anywhere in the body and is referred to by the location where it first appeared. For instance, breast cancer that begins in the breast and spreads to other parts of the body is still referred to as breast cancer. However, there are two main categories of cancer: **Hematologic (blood) cancers;** these are cancers of the blood cells, including leukemia, lymphoma, and multiple myeloma, while; **Solid tumor cancers** are cancers of any other organ, tissue or part of the body. The four most prevalent solid tumors are breast, prostate, lung, and colorectal. There are similarities between these cancers, but their growth, spread, and response to treatment may vary. Some cancers grow and spread rapidly, while others do so at a slower rate. Some are more likely to spread to other parts of the body, whereas others tend to remain in their original location.

A tumor is a lump or growth; it is an abnormal mass of tissue that surfaces when cells grow and divide abnormally or do not die when they should. Tumors or lumps that are not cancerous are referred to as benign, whereas cancerous lumps are referred to as malignant.

Cancer differs from benign tumors in that it can spread to other parts of the body, whereas benign tumors cannot. Cancer cells can break away from the origin of the disease. These cells can migrate to lymph nodes and other organs, where they can disrupt normal body functions.

TYPES OF CANCER

There exist numerous types of cancer and related hereditary syndromes, listed below are a few of them:

- Appendix Malignancy
- Breast carcinoma
- Bladder Cancer
- Bone Cancer
- Brain Tumour
- Prostate Cancer
- Colon Or Colorectal Cancer
- Duodenal Cancer
- Cancer of the ear
- Endometrial Cancer
- Oesophageal Malignancy
- Heart Disease
- Gallbladder Cancer
- Renal Or Kidney Cancer
- Laryngeal Malignancy
- Leukemia
- Mouth Cancer
- Lung cancer

- Lymphoma
- Mesothelioma
- Myeloma
- Ovarian carcinoma
- Pancreatic Malignancy
- Penile Cancer
- Rectal Cancer
- Skin disease
- Small Intestine Cancer
- Spleen Cancer
- Gastric Or Abdominal Cancer
- Testicular Cancer
- Thyroid Disease
- Uterine Cancer
- Cancer of the Vaginal and Vulvar Organs

Although we know more about some cancers than others, in the majority of cases we do not know why or how normal cells become cancerous. We are aware that changes occur in a series of steps, which typically take a considerable amount of time. The time between the first cell change and the detection of cancer is known as the latency period.

HOW CANCER SPREAD

It is possible for cancer to spread from the primary site to other parts of the body. When cancer cells break away from a tumor, they can spread through the bloodstream or lymph system.

Blood-borne cancer cells have the potential to reach distant organs. If cancer cells travel through the lymphatic system, they may end up in lymph nodes. In either case, the majority of escaped cancer cells die or are eliminated before they can begin to grow elsewhere. However, one or two cells may settle in a new location, begin to multiply, and form new tumors. This spread of cancer to a new location in the body is known as metastasis.

The cells of metastasis are identical to those of the primary cancer; they are not a new type of cancer. For example, breast cancer cells that have spread to the lungs are still breast cancer cells and NOT lung cancer cells, while colon cancer cells that have spread to the liver are still colon cancer cells.

Before cancer cells can spread to new parts of the body, they must undergo a series of transformations. They must first be able to detach from the primary tumor and then adhere to the exterior wall of a lymph vessel or blood vessel. Then, they must pass through the vessel wall in order to travel with the blood or lymph to a new organ or lymph node. Normal cells adhere to one another more strongly than cancer cells do. Additionally, they may produce substances that stimulate movement.

Cancer cells do not respond to signals indicating it is time for them to die, so they continue to divide and multiply rapidly. And they are adept at evading the immune system. When cancer cells remain in the tissue where they originated, this condition is known as carcinoma in situ (CIS).

Once these cells breach the tissue membrane, the condition is referred to as invasive cancer. Where cancer cells will spread next depends on their location in the body, but it is likely that they will spread in the immediate vicinity first. Cancer can spread by means of:

Tissue: A growing tumor can invade neighboring tissues or organs. Cancer cells can break away from the primary tumor and form new tumors nearby.

Spread through the bloodstream: Solid tumors require oxygen and other nutrients to thrive and spread via the bloodstream. During the process of Angiogenesis, tumors can induce the formation of new blood vessels to ensure their survival. Cancer cells are able to enter tiny blood vessels and then the bloodstream. These cells are known as circulating tumor cells (or CTCs).

Blood circulation sweeps cancer cells along until they become entrapped. Frequently, they become lodged in a capillary or other tiny blood vessel. The cancer cell must then pass through the capillary wall and into the tissue of the adjacent organ, then; the cell can proliferate and form a new tumor if:

- The conditions are favorable for its growth.
- It contains the necessary nutrients.

This is a fairly complex process, and the majority of cancer cells do not survive it. Only a handful of the tens of thousands of cancer cells that reach the bloodstream survive to form secondary cancers. Our immune system's white blood cells detect and kill some cancer cells.

Other cancer cells may perish as a result of the agitation caused by the rapid blood flow. Cancer cells in the bloodstream may attempt to clump together with platelets to protect themselves. Platelets are blood cells that contribute to blood clotting. This could also facilitate the spread of cancer cells into the surrounding tissues.

Spread through the lymphatic system: The lymphatic system is a collection of glands and tubes in the body responsible for filtering body fluid and fighting infection. Additionally, it captures damaged or malignant cells, such as cancer cells. Cancer cells can enter the lymph vessels close to the primary tumor and spread to the lymph glands or nodes in the area. In lymph glands, cancer cells may perish, however; some cells may survive and develop into tumors in one or more lymph nodes and this is known as lymph node spread.

Micro-metastases: These are areas of cancer spread that are too small to be observed, hence; they are hardly detected by any scan. Blood tests can detect certain proteins that cancer cells release; these proteins are sometimes referred to as tumor markers. However, there is no blood test that can determine whether a cancer has spread for the majority of cancers.

WHERE CANCER CAN SPREAD TO

Cancer cells have the ability to break off and spread through the blood or lymphatic systems to almost any part of the body. However, the majority of cancers tend to spread to one or two organs or parts of the body.

The pulmonary system: Lungs are the organ to which cancer most frequently spreads. This is because blood flows back to the heart and then to the lungs from the majority of the body parts. Cancer cells that entered the bloodstream can become trapped in the capillaries (small blood vessels) of the lungs. If cancer spreads to the lungs, you may exhibit no symptoms, or it may cause: persistent coughing, shortness of breath, chest infections, etc.

A pleural effusion is a build-up of fluid between the chest wall and the lung that can cause shortness of breath, chest pain, and discomfort. Cancer cells can cause inflammation in the two layers of tissue that cover the lungs (the pleural membrane), when this happens, fluid accumulates. Inflamed tissues produce excess fluid, which collects between membranes. Additionally, cancer cells in the pleural space may prevent the drainage of excess fluid. The lungs enlarge (inflate) when we inhale, this fluid accumulation obstructs and presses on the lungs, preventing them from fully expanding. Cancer that has spread to the lung (secondary lung cancer) is treated differently based on where the cancer originated in the body (primary cancer).

The Liver: Numerous forms of cancer can spread to the liver; however, it occurs most frequently in digestive system cancers. This is due to the fact that blood from the digestive system passes through the liver before returning to the heart, hence; the cancer cells may become trapped in the liver's capillaries. Cancer that has spread to the liver may not show any symptoms, but may result in:

- Fatigue, General malaise, Nausea, Appetite loss
- Pain under the right rib cage on the right side of the body
- Discoloration of the skin and eye whites (jaundice)
- Abdominal fluid accumulation (ascites)

Jaundice is caused by a blockage in the bile ducts or improper functioning of the liver, which can result in:

- The yellowish coloration of the skin and the sclera
- The skin becomes itchy
- Dark and pale coloration of urine and feces.

Ascites refers to an accumulation of fluid in the abdominal region. The abdomen contains numerous organs, including the stomach, intestines, and liver. These organs of the body are enclosed by a sheet of a membrane known as peritoneum. This peritoneum consists of two layers, one of which lines the abdominal wall and the other of which envelops the organs. Occasionally, fluid can accumulate between the two layers, which can be extremely unpleasant. Cancer cells can irritate the lining of the abdomen, causing it to produce too much fluid. Lymph glands in the abdomen can become blocked, preventing fluid from draining properly.

The liver's inability to produce sufficient blood proteins causes fluid to leak from veins into the abdominal cavity.

The lymph nodes: It is common for cancer cells to spread from their original location in the body to nearby lymph nodes. This is because tissue fluid naturally circulates from the organs to the lymphatic system. This is distinct from having lymphatic system cancer, such as lymphoma. When cancer spreads to lymph nodes, they may swell if the lymph nodes are close to the skin's surface, such as in the neck or under the arm, and they may be visible. However, if the lymph nodes are located deeper within the body, only a scan can detect them. Cancer of the lymph nodes may be asymptomatic; however, swollen lymph nodes can obstruct the flow of tissue fluid. This can lead to swelling in the body parts affected.

The bones: Certain cancers like prostate cancer, breast cancer, and lung cancer may spread to the bones. The most frequent effects of secondary cancer in the bones are pains in the affected bones; weakness in the affected bones; and elevated blood calcium levels. As cancer cells multiply in the bone and press on nerves, you experience pain. By causing damage to the bone's normal structure, a growing tumor can erode its strength. This can increase the likelihood of bone fracture (a pathological fracture). Bone cells that are damaged can release calcium into the blood. Blood calcium levels that are too high can cause nausea, fatigue, drowsiness or confusion, etc. Extremely high levels of calcium in the blood can result in irritability, confusion, and unconsciousness.

The brain: Some types of cancer, such as lung cancer and breast cancer, can spread to the brain. Colon cancer, kidney cancer, melanoma, and other cancers can sometimes spread to the brain. The most common symptoms of cancer that have spread to the brain are headaches, nausea, etc. Because there is limited space for the brain within the skull, these symptoms occur. Cancer that grows in the brain causes an increase in pressure inside the skull known as **raised intracranial pressure.** Depending on which region of the brain the cancer is growing and the size of the tumor (or tumors) other symptoms may manifest.

The Skin: Occasionally, cancer cells can grow in the skin. After the primary skin cancer has been surgically removed, secondary cancer may develop on or near the scar. Or, secondary skin cancers can sometimes develop in other areas of the body. Without treatment, the affected area may expand and bleed or exude fluid; this is known as ulcerating cancer.

STAGES OF CANCER

After a cancer diagnosis, one of the initial steps is cancer staging. Staging provides an overview of what to expect and aids in determining the most effective treatment. Staging involves determining the size of the tumor and its potential spread. This information is crucial for selecting the most likely effective treatments. Additionally, staging information can help your doctor locate clinical trials for which you may qualify.

Staging helps provide a general prognosis based on the experiences of others diagnosed at the same stage. Statistics on survival rates are based on the stage at diagnosis. However, your outlook depends on a variety of other factors that your doctor will discuss with you. Let us delve deeper into the stages of cancer, their determination, and their significance.

TNM system

T stands for tumor, N for lymph nodes, and M for metastasis in the TNM system.
The structure of the TNM system is as follows:

Primary Tumor

TX: Nothing is known or can be measured about the primary tumor.
T0: The primary tumor cannot be identified.
Tis: Cancer cells are only found in the layer of cells from which they originated (in situ), and do not affect deeper layers.
T1, T2, T3, T4: Size of the tumor from smallest to largest.

Lymph Nodes

NX: There are no information or lymph nodes that are inaccessible.
N0: Cancer is not detected in lymph nodes nearby.
N1, N2, N3: Describes the size, location, or quantity of cancerous lymph nodes.

Metastasis

M0: It does not appear that cancer has spread.

M1: The cancer has spread to remote locations.

Numbered staging

The combined information from the TNM categories constitutes the overall stage. For instance, a T1, N0, M0 pancreatic cancer would be considered stage 1. These stages are also divided into lettered subcategories, such as stage 2B, for certain types of cancer. In general, numbers or roman numerals may be used to represent the stages:

Stage 0: Precancer or cancer that has not spread from its original site. This is also referred to as in situ.

Stage 1: The cancer is small and has not spread and is also referred to as localized.

Stage 2: The cancer has grown or pushed into surrounding tissue, or has spread locally.

Stage 3: The cancer has grown in size and may have spread to the lymph nodes.

Stage 4: The cancer has spread to distant tissues or organs at this stage. This is terminal cancer.

Using Roman digits:

Stage 0: There is no cancer only abnormal cells with the potential to develop into cancer. This is also known as in situ carcinoma.

Stage I: indicates that the cancer is localized and small. This is also known as cancer at an early stage.

Stages II and III: Cancers are larger and have spread to nearby tissues or lymph nodes.

Stage IV: Cancer has spread to other parts of the body at this stage. It is also known as advanced cancer or metastatic.

Blood cancers, lymphomas, and brain cancer each have their staging systems. However, they all inform you of the cancer's progression.

CHAPTER 2

Is Cancer A Genetic Disease, Cancer Carcinogens, Risk Factors, Children And Cancer

IS CANCER A GENETIC DISEASE?

Cancer development may be influenced by genetic variables. The genetic code of an individual instructs cells when to proliferate and die. Gene mutations can lead to incorrect instructions, which can result in cancer. In addition to influencing the creation of proteins by cells, genes also affect the production of proteins, which carry many of the instructions for cellular development and division. Some genes alter proteins that would ordinarily heal damaged cells, which can lead to cancer in the long run. If a parent possesses these genes, they may transmit the changed instructions to their children. Some genetic modifications occur after birth, with risk factors including smoking and sun exposure. Other alterations that can lead to cancer occur in the chemical signals that dictate how the body deploys or expresses particular genes.

Gene Mutation and Cancer

A mutation in a gene can direct a healthy cell to:

Permit rapid development: A mutation in a gene can instruct a cell to grow and divide more rapidly. This generates numerous additional cells with the same mutation.

Fail to prevent unrestrained cell proliferation. Normal cells know when to cease dividing, allowing for an optimal quantity of each type of cell. Cancer cells lack these signaling components (tumor suppressor genes) that inform them when to cease growth. A mutation in a tumor suppressor gene enables the proliferation and accumulation of cancer cells.

Make mistakes when Fixing DNA errors. DNA repair genes scan a cell's DNA for faults and correct them. A mutation in a DNA repair gene may prevent the correction of additional errors, leading to the development of malignant cells (cancer). These are the most prevalent mutations detected in cancer, however; other gene alterations can contribute to cancer development.

Gene mutations can develop for various reasons, including:

Gene mutations inherited at birth: It is possible to inherit a genetic mutation from your parents at birth. This mutant type causes a minor proportion of malignancies.

Gene mutations that arise postnatally: The majority of gene mutations occur after birth and are not inherited. Several factors, including smoking, radiation, viruses, cancer-causing chemicals (carcinogens), obesity, hormones, chronic inflammation, and lack of exercise, can trigger gene alterations.

Mutations in genes are common during normal cell growth, however, cells feature a mechanism that recognizes when an error has occurred and corrects it. Infrequently, when a mistake is overlooked, a cell may become malignant.

How Gene Mutations Interact With One Another

Cancer is not caused by one genetic alteration, rather; it combines the gene mutations you are born with and those you acquire throughout your life. For instance, inheriting a genetic mutation that predisposes you to cancer does not guarantee that you will develop cancer, instead, cancer may require one or more gene alterations. Your hereditary gene mutation may increase your susceptibility to developing cancer when exposed to a particular carcinogen. It is unclear how many mutations must accumulate for cancer to develop; it is likely that this number differs between cancer types. A person can inherit a susceptibility to a certain type of cancer. A physician would refer to this as an inherited cancer syndrome.

CANCER CARCINOGENS

There are lots of risk factors for cancer, including age, family history, viruses and germs, lifestyle (behaviours), and exposure to (touching, consuming, inhaling, or inhaling) toxic substances. More than one hundred thousand chemicals are utilized by Americans, and roughly one thousand new chemicals are developed yearly. These compounds can be found in meals, personal care products, packaging, prescription medications, and household and yard care items. Although some chemicals can be toxic, not all chemical contact poses a health risk.

Cancer risk factors include habits such as smoking, high alcohol consumption, occupational exposure to chemicals, radiation, and sun exposure, as well as some viruses and bacteria. When all of these risks are taken into account, the significance of chemical exposures in producing cancer is minimal and unclear at present. Scientists have a limited understanding of how exposure to the majority of chemicals causes cancer. Carcinogens are substances that are known to induce cancer. Contact with a carcinogen does not guarantee the development of cancer. It depends, among other things, on what you were exposed to, how often you were exposed, how much you were exposed to, the frequency with which you were exposed, and your overall health. In the late 1700s, a link between cancer and a chemical was discovered. A considerable number of chimney sweeps were diagnosed with scrotal cancer as a result of their exposure to soot, which contains compounds known as polycyclic aromatic hydrocarbons. Many more substances have now been discovered as recognized or probable carcinogens. The majority of what we know today about chemicals that cause cancer in people comes from workers who were exposed on the job.

One of the major scientific obstacles we have today is understanding which chemicals cause specific tumors. Every day, humans are exposed to trace levels of several substances, these routine exposures are typically insufficient to create health issues. Exposure to chemicals in the environment, at home, and at work may increase the risk of developing cancer.

Certain chemicals, including benzene, beryllium, asbestos, vinyl chloride, and arsenic, are known to cause cancer in humans. Cancer risk is proportional to the amount, duration, frequency, and timing of exposure to certain substances. A modest dose in the fetus, for instance, could be more dangerous than a small exposure in an adult. The genes inherited from one's parents also play a part. Some substances are known to cause cancer in animals, but their link to human cancer has not been shown. These compounds are sometimes referred to be probable human carcinogens since it is likely that they will cause cancer in people. As potential human carcinogens, chloroform, DDT, formaldehyde, and polychlorinated biphenyls (PCBs) are examples.

Effects of Chemical Exposure in the Human Body

The human body has defences against all types of potentially cancer-causing exposures. When something enters the body, it frequently undergoes a procedure that facilitates its usage or elimination. The term for this process is metabolism. Depending on how a chemical is digested or metabolized in the body, there are three categories of carcinogens: direct-acting carcinogens, procarcinogens, and synergistic carcinogens (cocarcinogens).

DNA damage in cells can result in cancer, nevertheless, cells may frequently repair DNA damage. If the damage is severe, the cells could perish. Unrepaired DNA damage can result in gene mutations or alterations, and specific gene mutations can cause cancer.

Given that cancer has a lengthy incubation period, it is difficult to determine which exposure, if any, may have caused a mutation.

Cancer Clusters

Since numerous cancers are prevalent diseases, they occur often in populations. We anticipate finding multiple cancer cases in every particular area or workplace. Because the majority of malignancies are recorded in national databases, we have a reasonable understanding of how many cases to anticipate in a given region over a given period. However, several cancer cases in a community might generate tremendous alarm among locals. People may think that there is a cancer cluster in their town if a number of individuals have the disease. They may also suspect that environmental factors are to blame.

A cancer cluster occurs when a greater number of patients in a specified geographic area are diagnosed with the same type of cancer or associated malignancies than would be expected over a given length of time. However, what looks to be a cluster may really reflect the predicted number of cancer cases in the group or region, or it may be the result of pure chance. For instance, mesothelioma is exclusively seen in people who have been exposed to asbestos; hence, numerous occurrences of mesothelioma have been discovered in communities with asbestos exposure. Clusters of cancer are uncommon, especially those associated with environmental exposure.

When a group of malignancies is connected to environmental exposure, the following conditions are typically present:

- Many more cases than predicted of one specific type of cancer or related cancers have been discovered.
- The cancer is found in an age range where it is uncommon.
- The type of cancer is uncommon.
- Scientific data confirms the link between the chemical in question and cancer.

It is difficult to determine how much a community has been exposed to a cancer-causing material. Many hazardous waste sites, for instance, include many chemicals, making it difficult to attribute health results to a particular chemical exposure.

RISK FACTORS

Over 180 distinct cancer kinds have been found owing to the numerous risk factors, including age, genetics, and lifestyle choices can increase your likelihood of developing cancer. Cancer is typically caused by a combination of multiple risk factors. The more predisposing factors you have, the greater your cancer risk. The most significant risk factors include:

Age: Cancer can affect people of all ages, but older people are at increased risk.

Genetics: Family history may increase one's cancer risk. If you or a member of your family has a certain type of cancer, you may be at a higher risk for developing that disease. Many cancers, including breast cancer and colon cancer, are strongly influenced by genetics.

Behaviours: Cancer risk factors include tobacco use and exposure to the sun or other sources of UV radiation. In addition, a bad diet, a lack of physical activity, and excessive alcohol consumption, other lifestyle choices may increase cancer risk.

Viruses or bacteria: Certain types of cancer are caused by viruses or bacteria. Human papillomavirus (HPV), which causes cervical cancer, hepatitis B and C viruses, which can cause liver cancer, and Epstein-Barr virus, which may cause a kind of lymphoma, are all viruses associated with cancer. Additionally, H. pylori can cause stomach cancer.

Chemical Exposures: As previously mentioned, exposure to chemicals may also be a predisposing factor.

Behavioural Risk Factors

The decisions you make about your lifestyle can reduce your risk of developing cancer. These include avoiding cigarette (tobacco) use and exposure to second-hand smoke, limiting alcohol intake, limiting exposure to sunlight and tanning beds, protecting oneself from sexually transmitted diseases, maintaining a healthy body weight, and engaging in regular physical activity.

Tobacco is responsible for thirty percent of all cancers. Cigarette, cigar, and pipe smoking can lead to lung, mouth, throat, larynx (voice box), esophagus, pancreas, kidney, bladder, stomach, and cervical cancers, in addition to acute myeloid leukemia.

You should also avoid second-hand smoke, which causes lung cancer in individuals who do not smoke and may increase the risk of other cancers in adults and children.

Diet & Exercise: Maintain a healthy weight and a physically active lifestyle. Obesity increases the risk of developing breast, colon, kidney, and esophageal cancers. Physical activity may help reduce the risk of certain malignancies, including colon and breast cancers.

Sexual Behaviour: Certain strains of HPV cause cervical, vaginal, and other genital malignancies. Sexual contact spreads genital HPV, however using a condom may minimize your risk of contracting the virus. Vaccines can prevent infections with some cancer-causing HPV strains, but not all.

Alcohol: Excessive alcohol consumption may increase the risk of developing cancer. Long-term alcohol consumption is connected with oral, pharyngeal, esophageal, liver, colon, and breast cancers.

Medical Examinations and Treatments: Certain medical tests, such as imaging scans, can raise the risk of developing cancer. In women, hormones and hormone-related medicines, such as menopausal hormone therapy, may raise their chance of developing breast or uterine cancer. Even some cancer therapies, like medications and radiation, have been shown to raise the patient's risk of developing cancer again. Discuss the risks and advantages of medical testing and treatments with your doctor.

Exposure in the Workplace: Although everyday chemical exposures are typically too low to create health problems, exposure in the workplace can be more hazardous. Chemical exposures in the workplace can occur at high concentrations and over extended periods. Consequently, some tasks necessitate the use of protective gear, equipment, and/or respirators, hence; companies are required to inform their employees of any health risks. Remember that job exposure to hazardous substances might vary significantly from exposure in other situations.

Pollution and Chemical Exposure: Exposure to harmful chemicals and substances can raise the risk of cancer. Asbestos, nickel, cadmium, radon, vinyl chloride, benzidene, and benzene are well-known carcinogens. These carcinogens may increase your risk alone or in conjunction with another carcinogen. For instance, asbestos workers who also smoke are more likely to develop lung cancer.

CHILDREN AND CANCER

The reason for which children develop cancer is particularly challenging to comprehend and accept. Before the age of 15, cancer will be diagnosed in approximately 1 in 450 youngsters. The majority of juvenile malignancies have unclear causes. Unlike adult cancers, children's cancers are mostly unrelated to lifestyle-related risk factors. Childhood malignancies are associated with genetic susceptibility (family history), radiation exposure, infections and illnesses, prenatal health concerns, and chemical exposure.

Some experts believe that mutated cells in the quickly developing body of a child divide before their DNA can be repaired. This could contribute to the occurrence of paediatric cancer.

Stem cells, which are simple cells capable of generating various types of specialized cells that the body requires, are frequently the site of childhood malignancies or their origin. Typically, a random (happens by chance) cell alteration or mutation causes juvenile cancer. In adults, epithelial cells typically transform into malignant cells. Epithelial cells line the body's inside and cover its exterior. Over time, environmental exposures to these cells cause cancer. For this reason, adult cancers are sometimes referred to as acquired. Children and adults can develop cancer in the same areas of the body, but there are variances. There is a high percentage of remission for childhood malignancies, which can come unexpectedly and without warning signs. Leukemia is the most frequent form of cancer among children. Additional childhood cancers include brain tumors, lymphoma, and soft tissue sarcoma.

The prognosis, diagnosis, and treatment of childhood cancers differ from those of adult tumors. The primary distinctions are the survival rate and the cancer's etiology (cause). The five-year survival rate for children cancer is approximately 80%, compared to 68% for adult cancers. It is believed that paediatric cancer is more sensitive to treatment and that children can withstand more aggressive treatments.

CHAPTER 3

Finding Or Diagnosing Cancer, Signs and Symptoms, Treatments For Cancer, Possible Complications, Preventive Measures

FINDING OR DIAGNOSING CANCER

Efficient diagnostic testing is utilized to confirm or rule out the presence of disease, monitor the progression of the disease, and assess the efficacy of treatment. If a person's health has changed, if the sample collected was of poor quality, or if an aberrant test result needs to be confirmed, it may be essential to repeat testing.

A greater number of people are surviving cancer as a result of earlier identification and, more effective treatment options. Screening is the process of detecting cancer before symptoms appear. Regular screening may detect breast, cervical, and colorectal cancers in their earliest, most treatable stages. Imaging, laboratory tests (including tests for tumor markers), tumor biopsy, endoscopic examination, surgery, and genetic testing are among the diagnostic procedures for cancer.

Laboratory Test: Clinical chemistry utilizes chemical methods to measure the concentrations of chemical components in bodily fluids and tissues. Blood and urine are the most common specimens utilized in clinical chemistry. Numerous assays exist to identify and quantify virtually any chemical component in blood or urine.

These components include blood glucose, electrolytes, enzymes, hormones, lipids (fats), other metabolic components, and proteins.

The following are examples of frequent laboratory tests:

- Blood testing
- Total blood cell count (CBC)
- Urinalysis
- Tumor markers

Diagnostic Imaging: In recent years, diagnostic radiology has made enormous strides with the development of new devices and techniques that can identify cancer more accurately and help patients avoid surgery. Imaging is the technique of creating images of valuable biological structures and organs. It is utilized to detect cancers and other abnormalities, ascertain the extent of disease, and assess the efficacy of treatment. Additionally, imaging may be utilized for doing biopsies and other surgical procedures. There are three imaging techniques utilized for cancer diagnosis: transmission imaging, reflection imaging, and emission imaging; each employs a distinct method.

- **Transmission imaging:** Computed tomography (CT) scans, X-rays, fluoroscopy, and other radiological procedures generate images via transmission. In transmission imaging, a high-energy photon beam is created and passes through the studied body structure.

The X-ray beam swiftly passes through less dense types of tissue, such as watery fluids, blood, and fat, leaving a darker region on the film. Gray is the color of muscle and connective tissues (ligaments, tendons, and cartilage), while the bones will look white.

- **Reflection imaging:** Reflection imaging is the imaging created by transmitting high-frequency sounds to the observed body region or organ. Depending on the tissue density, these sound waves "bounce" off the various types of biological tissues and structures at varying speeds. The reflected sound waves are transmitted to a computer, which analyses the sound waves and generates a visual image of the bodily part or structure; for example, ultrasound.

- **Emission imaging:** Emission imaging occurs when a scanner detects and analyses small nuclear particles or magnetic energy to produce an image of the inspected body structure or organ. Nuclear medicine employs the emission of radioactive particles from radioactive substances put into the body for examination. Using radio waves and a piece of equipment that generates a strong magnetic field, magnetic resonance imaging (MRI) induces cells to produce their own radio frequencies.

Endoscopic Examinations: An endoscope is a portable, flexible tube equipped with a light and a lens that is used to examine the esophagus, stomach, duodenum, colon, or rectum. A probe at the end of the endoscope is utilized to bounce high-energy sound waves (ultrasound) off the interior organs in order to create an image (sonogram).

It can also be used to remove tissue from the body for screening and to picture the interior of the body in color.
Endoscopic types include:
- Sigmoidoscopy
- Retrograde endoscopic cholangiopancreatography (ERCP)
- Cystoscopy (also called cystourethroscopy)
- Esophagogastroduodenoscopy (also called EGD or upper endoscopy)
- Colonoscopy

Genetic Testing: This test is designed to identify inherited gene mutations that may increase a person's chance of developing certain types of cancer. This is accomplished by searching for specific alterations in your genes, chromosomes, or proteins. These modifications are known as mutations. There are genetic testing available for numerous forms of cancer. It is difficult to detect mutations in genes that raise the risk of cancer. Understanding these principles is essential when contemplating cancer susceptibility gene testing.

Tumor Biopsies: A small tissue sample is taken surgically and analyzed under a microscope for the presence of cancer cells. Depending on the location of the tumor, certain biopsies can be performed in the outpatient setting using just a local anesthetic. Fluid-filled tumors are biopsied using a technique called fine needle aspiration. A long, thin needle is immediately placed into the questionable location to withdraw fluid samples for analysis.

Blood levels of tumor markers (substances produced into the bloodstream by specific tumors) may provide additional evidence for or against the diagnosis of cancer when examination findings or imaging test results imply cancer. Tumor markers may be useful for monitoring the efficacy of treatment and detecting the likely recurrence of cancer in patients who have been diagnosed with specific types of cancer. For certain malignancies, the level of a tumor marker decreases during therapy and rises if the cancer returns. Some tumor markers are not detectable in the blood but are present in tumor cells. These indicators are identified by analyzing a biopsy sample of tissue.

Typically, biopsies are conducted to assess if a tumor is malignant (cancerous) or to identify the source of an inexplicable illness or inflammation.

These are the most frequent forms of biopsies:
- Endoscopic biopsy
- Bone marrow biopsy
- Excisional or incisional tissue sampling
- Biopsy via fine needle aspiration
- Punch biopsy
- Shave pathology
- Skin biopsy

Ultrasound, X-ray, CT, and MRI are all harmless and non-invasive; but, because too many CT and x-rays expose you to radiation, they can raise your risk of acquiring cancer. In the majority of instances, its benefits outweigh the hazards.

Mammograms are one use of X-ray technology that may be utilized in the process of cancer detection. Pap screenings, that look for abnormal cervical cells; HPV DNA tests, that further look for DNA from cancer-causing HPV types in cervical cells; faecal occult blood tests (FOBT), which evaluate for blood in the stool; sigmoidoscopy, which observes the lower colon; and colonoscopy, which examines the entire colon are other methods for detecting and diagnosing cancer or abnormal cells that may develop into cancer.

SIGNS AND SYMPTOMS

Signs and symptoms are the manners in which the body alerts you to an accident, illness, or disease. Cancer symptoms vary on the cancer's location, its size, and the extent to which it affects neighboring organs or tissues. If a cancer has spread (metastasized), signs and symptoms may manifest in several bodily locations. Symptoms of cancer may also include fever, excessive exhaustion, and weight loss. This may be because cancer cells consume a significant amount of the body's energy. Or, cancer may produce molecules that alter how the body generates energy. Additionally, cancer can cause the immune system to react in ways that elicit similar symptoms.

The majority of signs and symptoms are not caused by cancer, but rather by other conditions. If you experience persistent or worsening signs and symptoms, you should visit a doctor to determine the cause. If cancer is not the reason, a doctor can assist determine and treat the underlying problem.

Lymph nodes, for instance, are part of the body's immune system that assist trap dangerous chemicals. Normal lymph nodes are minute and difficult to locate. However, when there is an infection, inflammation, or malignancy, the lymph nodes might swell. Those near the skin's surface can become large enough to be felt, and some can even be visible as a bulge or a lump beneath the skin. One cause of lymph node enlargement is the presence of cancer cells. Therefore, if you have an odd lump or swelling, you should visit your doctor to determine the cause. However; here are some of the most prevalent cancer-related signs and symptoms, but note that any of them might also be caused by other issues.

Abnormal pelvic pain or periods: Majority of women experience irregular periods or cramps occasionally. However, prolonged discomfort or a change in your menstrual cycle may indicate cervical, uterine, or ovarian cancer.

Bathroom habit changes: Significant changes in body functions may suggest malignancies such as colon, prostate, and bladder. Constipation or diarrhea that persists, black or red blood in the stool, black, tarry stools, increased urination, and blood in the urine are indicators of colorectal cancer.

Bloating: Everyone occasionally feels bloated, but bloating lasting more than two weeks might be an indication of ovarian cancer and other gastrointestinal malignancies.

Changes in the Breast: These include a new lump, dimpling, discoloration, changes around the nipple, or an unusual discharge. Although breast cancer is more prevalent in women, men can still acquire the disease.

Chronic cough or hoarseness: A cough that lingers for more than two weeks, particularly a dry cough, may be an indication of lung cancer, whereas hoarseness may indicate cancer of the larynx or thyroid.

Persistent headache: Brain tumors can produce headaches that persist longer than two weeks and do not respond to conventional treatments.

Swallowing difficulties: If you feel food becoming caught in your throat or have difficulty swallowing for more than two weeks, this might be an indication of throat, lung, or stomach cancer.

Excessive bruising: A bruise on the shin caused by a collision with the coffee table is typical. However, a rapid increase in the number of bruises in strange locations that have not been bumped might suggest a variety of blood malignancies.

Frequent fevers or infections: A recurrent fever or a progression from one illness to the next may suggest that lymphoma or leukemia has weakened the immune system.

Oral alterations: Persistent sores, lesions, or painful places in the mouth, particularly in heavy smokers or drinkers, might suggest a variety of oral malignancies.

Persistent fatigue: A rapid, long-lasting shift in your energy level, regardless of how much sleep you have been receiving, may indicate leukemia or lymphoma, or you may experience blood loss due to colon or stomach malignancy. Consult a physician if rest does not alleviate your fatigue.

Postmenopausal bleeding: There are several causes for this, but if it prolongs, your doctor may check for cervical or uterine cancer.

Abdominal pain or nausea: Pain that persists for more than two weeks may be an indicator of liver, pancreas, or other digestive system malignancies.

Unexplained weight loss: Nearly half of cancer patients lose weight. It is typically one of the first indicators they detect. Unintentional weight loss or loss of appetite can be indicative of a variety of malignancies, especially those that have spread.

Unusual lumps: Any persistent new lump or mass should be investigated. When you have a cold, lymph nodes frequently expand, but if the swelling remains after you recover, you should visit your doctor.

Pain. Bone cancers frequently cause pain from the start. Some brain tumors result in daily headaches that do not respond to therapy. Additionally, pain might be a late symptom of certain types of malignancies.

Skin changes: Unusual or new moles, lumps, or markings on your body are likely indicators of skin cancer.

Your skin might also reveal indications of other types of cancer. It might be an indication of liver, ovarian, or kidney cancer or lymphoma if it becomes darker, becomes yellow or red, itchy, grows more hair, or if you have an inexplicable rash.

Wounds that fail to heal. Bleeding and persistent spots are also indicators of skin cancer. Oral ulcers can be the first sign of oral cancer. If you smoke, chew tobacco, or consume excessive amounts of alcohol, your risk is increased.

Unexplained bleeding: Cancer can cause blood to appear in inappropriate places. Blood in faeces is an indication of colon or rectal cancer. Additionally, malignancies in the urinary canal might lead to blood in the urine.

Anemia: This occurs when the body lacks sufficient red blood cells, which are produced in the bone marrow. Cancers such as leukemia, lymphoma, and multiple myeloma can cause marrow destruction. Red blood cells may be crowded out by tumors that have spread there from other locations.

Extremely excessive night-time perspiration: Night-time perspiration can be caused by illnesses or be a side effect of some drugs. It is also commonly experienced by women throughout menopause. However, extremely heavy, drenching night sweats may potentially indicate malignancy.

Problems urinating: A enlarged prostate might make it difficult to urinate or cause you to urinate often. Inform your doctor if you have urinary discomfort or detect blood in your urine.

A bulge, discomfort, or aching in the scrotum. This may indicate testicular cancer.

Vaginal bleeding or discharge: Get screened if it happens between periods or after menopause. Endometrial cancer can cause unexpected bruising and bleeding.

Appetite changes: Ovarian cancer might make you feel full or make eating difficult. Other malignancies can induce nausea or indigestion. Cancer is not the only disease that can alter your appetite, but if you have had problems eating for two weeks or longer, consult your doctor.

Note, aside from the above-listed symptoms and or signs; there are several other health issues cancer can induce, ensure you consult a physician when such issues persist.

TREATMENTS FOR CANCER

The objective of cancer treatment is to achieve a cure for a particular kind of cancer, thereby enabling the patient to live a healthy lifespan. Depending on your unique situation, this may or may not be doable. If a cure is not possible, treatments may be used to decrease or slow the progression of your cancer so that you can live as long as possible symptom-free. Many cancer treatments are available, so; treatment options will be determined by a number of criteria, including the kind and stage of your cancer, your overall health condition, and your preferences. Depending on your specific circumstances, you may receive a single treatment or a mix of treatments.

Treatments for cancer may be used as:

Initial or Primary Treatment: The purpose of a primary treatment is to eradicate the cancer from the body or to kill all cancer cells. Any cancer treatment can be used as a primary treatment, but surgery is the most common primary treatment for the most prevalent cancer types. If your cancer is especially susceptible to radiation therapy or chemotherapy, you may receive one of these treatments as your initial treatment.

Adjuvant Treatment: Adjuvant therapy aims to eliminate any remaining cancer cells after primary treatment in order to reduce the likelihood of cancer recurrence. As an adjuvant therapy, any cancer treatment may be used. Chemotherapy, radiation therapy, and hormone therapy are common adjuvant therapies. Similar to adjuvant therapy, neoadjuvant therapies are administered before the primary treatment to make it easier or more successful.

Palliative Treatment: Palliative therapy may alleviate treatment-related adverse effects or cancer-related signs and symptoms. Surgery, radiation, chemotherapy, and hormone therapy are all viable options for symptom relief. Pain and shortness of breath may be alleviated by further drugs. Palliative treatment can be administered along with other cancer-curing therapies.

Options for cancer treatment include:

Surgery: The purpose of surgery is to eliminate all or as much cancer as feasible.

Chemotherapy: Chemotherapy refers to the employment of medications to eradicate cancer cells. The medications may be administered orally or intravenously. Different types of medications may be administered simultaneously or sequentially.

Radiation Treatment: To eradicate cancer cells, radiation therapy employs high-powered energy beams, such as X-rays or protons. Cancer cells proliferate and divide more rapidly than healthy cells. Because radiation is most damaging to rapidly dividing cells, radiation therapy is more detrimental to cancer cells than to normal ones. This inhibits the growth and division of cancer cells, resulting in cell death. Two main types of radiation therapy exist:

- **External beam:** This is the most widespread form. It intends to use x-rays or particles to identify the tumor externally.
- **Internal beam**: This kind emits radiation within the body. It may be administered via radioactive seeds implanted into or near the tumor, an oral liquid or pill, or intravenously (intravenous, or IV).

Bone Marrow Transplantation: Bone marrow is the tissue within bones that produces blood cells from blood stem cells. A bone marrow transplant, also known as a stem cell transplant, can employ either your own or a donor's stem cells.

A bone marrow transplant enables your doctor to treat your cancer with stronger doses of chemotherapy. Additionally, it can be utilized to replace damaged bone marrow.

Immunotherapy: Immunotherapy is a cancer treatment that depends on the body's ability to fight infection (immune system). It uses molecules produced by the body or in a laboratory to assist the immune system in working harder or more precisely against cancer. This assists the body in eliminating cancer cells. Immunotherapy operates via:

- Stopping or reducing cancer cell growth
- Preventing the spread of cancer to other areas of the body
- Improving the ability of the immune system to eliminate cancer cells

These drugs are designed to target specific cancer cell components. Some have attached toxins or radioactive substances. Immunotherapy is administered intravenously.

Hormone Therapy: This is used to treat cancers like breast, prostate, and ovarian that are fuelled by hormones. It uses surgery or medications to stop or block the production of the body's natural hormones. This helps to inhibit the expansion of cancer cells. The surgery involves removing hormone-producing organs, such as the ovaries or testes. The drugs are administered intravenously or orally.

Targeted drug therapy: In targeted drug therapy, medications are used to prevent the growth and spread of cancer. It accomplishes this with less damage to normal cells than competing therapies.

Standard chemotherapy kills cancer cells as well as some healthy ones. Targeted therapy focuses on specific targets (molecules) within cancer cells. These targets play a role in the growth and survival of cancer cells. By inhibiting these targets, the medication renders cancer cells incapable of spreading. Targeted treatment medications function in a variety of ways. They may: Stop the process in cancer cells that leads them to develop and spread; Induce cancer cells to die on their own; Directly kill cancer cells.

Cryoablation. This treatment utilizes cold to eliminate cancer cells. During cryoablation, a thin, wand-like needle (cryoprobe) is introduced directly into the malignant tumor via the skin. The cryoprobe is pumped with a gas to freeze the tissue. The tissue is then permitted to defrost. In order to eradicate cancer cells, the freezing and thawing process is performed multiple times within the same therapy session.

Ablation with radiofrequency energy: This treatment uses electrical energy to heat and kill cancer cells. A doctor guides a tiny needle through the skin or an incision and into the cancerous tissue during radiofrequency ablation. By passing high-frequency energy through the needle, the surrounding tissue is heated, thereby destroying the neighboring cells.

Laser Therapy: Laser therapy destroys cancer cells using a very narrow, focused beam of light. Laser treatment is useful for:

- Eliminate malignant and precancerous growths.
- Reduce the size of tumors obstructing the stomach, colon, or esophagus.
- Treat symptoms of cancer, such as bleeding.
- After surgery, seal nerve ends to decrease discomfort.
- Seal lymph vessels following surgery to minimize edema and prevent the spread of malignant cells.

Laser therapy is frequently administered using a tiny, illuminated tube inserted into the body. At the end of the tube, thin fibers steer light toward cancer cells. Lasers are utilized on the skin as well. Most frequently, lasers are combined with other cancer treatments, such as radiation and chemotherapy.

Photodynamic Therapy: A patient is injected with a medication that is sensitive to a certain type of light in photodynamic therapy. The medication remains longer in cancer cells than in healthy cells. The physician then focuses light from a laser or other source on the cancer cells. The light converts the medication into a chemical that destroys cancer cells.

Cryotherapy: This technique, also known as cryosurgery, employs extremely cold gas to freeze and kill cancer cells. On the skin or cervix, for instance, it is occasionally used to treat cells that could become malignant (termed precancerous cells). Doctors can also use a specialized device to provide cryotherapy to internal tumors, such as those in the liver or prostate. Depending on the type of cancer, other treatments may be possible.

POSSIBLE COMPLICATIONS

Numerous cancer patients are susceptible to having long-term adverse effects. These adverse effects may occur months or years following treatment. Evaluation and treatment of late effects are essential components of cancer survivorship care. Side effects might vary from person to person, as well as between medications and treatments. Listed below are the most prevalent adverse effects.

Neutropenia: Neutropenia is a decrease in white blood cells, the body's primary defence against infection. Neutropenia is prevalent following chemotherapy treatment. Chemotherapy medications eliminate rapidly dividing cells in the body, including cancer cells and healthy white blood cells. During chemotherapy, your white blood cell count may be lower than normal, making you more susceptible to infection.

Lymphedema: If lymph nodes are removed during surgery or if a lymph node or lymph vessel is damaged by radiation therapy, the lymph fluid may not drain adequately. The accumulation of fluid under your skin may cause a portion of your body to bulge. This disorder is known as lymphedema.

Hair Loss: Certain types of chemotherapy might cause hair loss. This disorder is known as alopecia. Typically, hair regrows two to three months after therapy ends. A cooling cap could help you retain more hair. A cooling cap fits snugly and keeps your scalp cool before, during, and after chemotherapy. According to studies, the effectiveness of a cooling cap relies on the type of chemotherapy administered.

Nausea and Vomiting: Immunotherapy, radiation therapy to the abdomen, and chemotherapy are all known to produce nausea and vomiting in cancer patients (with results ranging by medication type and dose). Nausea and vomiting might result in weight fluctuations, dehydration, and malnutrition, which can exacerbate the side effects. Thankfully, medications can help decrease nausea and improve your condition. Additionally, nausea can be treated in different ways, intake of fluid like water or ginger ale may help. Some people utilize relaxation techniques, hypnosis, or acupuncture.

Difficulty Concentrating and Recalling Information: Some individuals may experience difficulty concentrating or recalling information as a side effect of cancer treatments. This is sometimes referred to as "chemo brain," and it can make it difficult for cancer patients to perform their jobs or daily duties. Tips for dealing with this issue include getting enough sleep, writing down your daily goals and putting reminders on your smartphone, and focusing on a single activity rather than attempting to multitask.

Deep vein thrombosis (DVT): This is the formation of a blood clot in a deep vein. Typically, these clots originate in the lower leg, thigh, or pelvis, although they can also form in the arm. Occasionally, the DVT can break off and travel to the lungs. Cancer patients, especially those receiving chemotherapy, have a significantly increased risk of DVT compared to the general population.

High Blood Pressure (Hypertension): This may occur in conjunction with CHF (Congestive heart failure) or as a distinct symptom. If you have hypertension, your physician may monitor it more closely throughout cancer therapy. Accelerated hypertension is characterized by a sudden and rapid rise in blood pressure, which frequently results in organ damage; therefore, it is imperative to seek immediate medical attention. Examples of cancer medications that can lead to hypertension include Bevacizumab (Avastin, Mvasi); Sorafenib (Nexavar); Sunitinib (Sutent).

The risk of hypertension decreases as a person quits using these medications. However, the long-term consequences are unknown. Survivors at greater risk for hypertension should collaborate with their health care team to reduce this risk. This may involve measuring blood pressure, lowering weight, reducing salt intake, taking medication, and engaging in physical activity.

Heart Problems: Both chemotherapy and chest radiation therapy can produce cardiac complications. Some cancer survivors may be at an increased risk, this includes those who:

- Received Hodgkin lymphoma treatment as a youngster
- Are 65 and older
- Received greater chemotherapy dosages
- Obtained specific medications, including trastuzumab (Herceptin, Ogivri) and doxorubicin (Adriamycin, Doxil)

Listed below are common heart problems. Consult your physician immediately if you experience any of the following symptoms:

- Congestive heart failure (CHF) is cardiac muscle deterioration. Symptoms include shortness of breath, disorientation, and hand or foot swelling.

- Coronary artery disease is a form of cardiovascular disease. Those who have had significant doses of radiation therapy to the chest are particularly susceptible. Chest pain and shortness of breath are symptoms.

- Arrhythmia is a heartbeat that is irregular. Among the symptoms include dizziness, chest pain, and shortness of breath.

Examples of medicines that can induce cardiovascular issues: Trastuzumab, Doxorubicin, Daunorubicin (Cerubidine), Epirubicin (Ellence), The drug Cyclophosphamide (Genoxal, Mitoxan), Osemertinib (Tagrisso) (Tagrisso).

Ask your physician if the medications you are taking can impact your heart. During and after therapy, he or she may monitor your heart function and look for any signs of damage.

Lung issues. Chest chemotherapy and radiation therapy may harm the lungs. Survivors of cancer who have received both chemotherapy and radiation therapy may be at an increased risk for lung damage. People with a history of lung disease and older adults may be more susceptible to lung difficulties.

The following drugs may cause lung damage:

- Bleomycin (Blexane) (Blexane)
- Carmustine (Becenum, BiCNU, Carmubris) (Becenum, BiCNU, Carmubris)
- The drug Methotrexate (multiple brand names)

The lung's late consequences may include:

- A change in the pulmonary function
- Thickening of the pulmonary lining
- Pneumonia is characterized by inflammation of the lungs
- Difficulty in respiration

Endocrine system problems: Certain forms of cancer treatments may cause difficulties with the endocrine system. This system contains the glands and organs that produce hormones and eggs or sperm. Cancer survivors who are at risk for hormone changes as a result of treatment must undergo routine blood testing to assess hormone levels.

Bone, joint, and soft tissue conditions: Chemotherapy, corticosteroid medicines, and hormone therapy can cause osteoporosis and joint pain. Immunotherapy may result in joint or muscle issues. These are referred to as rheumatologic conditions. People who are inactive may be at a greater risk for these illnesses. In the following strategies, cancer survivors might reduce their risk of osteoporosis by:

- Refraining from using tobacco goods
- Consuming dietary sources of calcium and vitamin D
- Engaging in physical activity
- Limiting their alcohol consumption

Issues with the brain, spinal cord, and nerves. The brain, spinal cord, and nerves may have long-term negative effects after chemotherapy and radiation therapy. These consist of:

- Hearing loss caused by large doses of chemotherapy, particularly cisplatin (multiple brand names).
- Increased risk of stroke due to high brain radiation doses
- Adverse effects on the nervous system, including nerve damage outside the brain and spinal cord.

After treatment, cancer survivors should undergo routine physical examinations and hearing tests to check for these side effects. Depending on the therapies they got, cancer survivors may experience dental and oral health issues, as well as visual problems. Chemotherapy may negatively impact tooth enamel and raise the risk of long-term dental issues. Radiation therapy to the head and neck at high dosages may alter tooth development. Additionally, it might promote gum disease and reduce saliva production, resulting in a dry mouth. Steroid medicines may raise the likelihood of developing eye issues. This includes cataracts, a clouding of the eye that impairs vision. Survivors should plan monthly check-ups with a dentist and an ophthalmologist to monitor for any complications.

Chemotherapy, radiation therapy, and surgery may impact a person's ability to digest food. Abdominal surgery or radiation therapy can result in scarring, chronic pain, and intestinal complications. Some survivors may develop chronic diarrhea, which hinders the body's absorption of nutrients.

A licensed dietitian (RD) can assist individuals with digestive issues in obtaining sufficient nutrients. Additionally, it may be good to see a gastroenterologist or a specialist in the digestive tract.

Emotional difficulties: Cancer survivors frequently experience a range of positive and negative feelings, including but not limited to fear of recurrence, anger, guilt, despair, anxiety, a sense of isolation, etc. Cancer survivors, caregivers, family members, and friends may acquire post-traumatic stress disorder after experiencing a terrifying or life-threatening experience, such as a cancer diagnosis or treatment. Each individual's post-treatment experience is unique.

Reoccurring Cancer or Secondary Cancer: It is possible that this may be a new primary cancer. It may occur as a late result of chemotherapy and radiation therapy used to treat cancer in the past. Or it could be the initial cancer that has spread to other areas of the body. Chemotherapy and radiation therapy can also harm stem cells in the bone marrow. Either acute leukemia or myelodysplasia is more likely as a result. Myelodysplasia is a blood malignancy in which normal blood components are either absent or aberrant. Discuss with your physician any new symptoms or adverse effects you experience.

Fatigue is a persistent feeling of physical, emotional, or mental exhaustion. It is the most prevalent treatment-related adverse event. Some cancer survivors experience exhaustion months or even years after treatment has ended.

PREVENTIVE MEASURES

Probably, we have seen a number of contradictory reports regarding cancer prevention. Occasionally, a certain cancer preventive tip proposed by one study is discouraged by another. Frequently, cancer preventive knowledge is still evolving. However, it is widely acknowledged that your cancer risk is influenced by your lifestyle choices. Therefore, if you are concerned about preventing cancer, bear in mind that simple lifestyle modifications can make a difference. Consider these tips for cancer prevention:

Do not use tobacco products: In the United States, roughly 30% of all malignancies and 90% of lung cancers are caused by smoking. Approximately half of all smokers die from a smoking-related illness, such as cancer, heart disease, chronic obstructive pulmonary disease, mouth, throat, larynx, pancreas, bladder, cervix, and kidney. Tobacco causes over five million fatalities annually on a global scale and is estimated to cause one billion deaths by the end of the century. Chewing tobacco has been related to oral cavity and pancreatic cancer. Even if you do not use tobacco, passive smoking may raise your risk of developing lung cancer. Tobacco avoidance and cessation are crucial components of cancer prevention.

Consume a Healthy Diet: While choosing healthy foods at the grocery store and meals cannot ensure cancer prevention, it may lessen your risk.

Maintain a healthy weight by consuming fruits, vegetables, and other plant-based foods, such as whole grains and beans. Consume less high-calorie foods, particularly refined carbohydrates, and animal fat, in order to lose weight. Reduce your consumption of processed meats. The World Health Organization's cancer agency, the International Agency for Research on Cancer, determined in a report that consuming high quantities of processed beef may modestly raise the risk of developing some types of cancer.

In addition, a Mediterranean diet enriched with extra-virgin olive oil and mixed nuts may lessen the incidence of breast cancer in women. The majority of the Mediterranean diet consists of plant-based foods, such as fruits and vegetables, whole grains, legumes, and nuts. People who adhere to the Mediterranean diet favour healthy fats like olive oil over butter and fish over red meat.

Maintaining a healthy weight and engaging in physical activity: Maintaining a healthy weight reduces the risk of certain types of cancer, such as breast, prostate, lung, colon, and kidney cancer. The manner in which weight increases cancer risk differs by cancer. For instance, estrogen produced by fat cells likely increases the risk of postmenopausal breast cancer; blood sugar and insulin problems associated with obesity likely increase the risk of colon and pancreatic cancer; and weight-related irritations caused by gallstones and acid reflux likely increase the risk of cancers of the gallbladder and esophagus, respectively.

The increasingly well-known and alarming increases in the incidence of overweight and obesity in the United States foretell a growing burden of weight-related malignancies as well as cardiovascular disease, stroke, and diabetes.

Physical activity also counts, in addition to assisting with weight management, physical activity may reduce the risk of breast and colon cancer. Adults who engage in any level of physical activity receive health benefits. However, for major health advantages, aim for at least 150 minutes of moderate aerobic activity per week or 75 minutes of vigorous aerobic activity per week. Include at least 30 minutes of physical activity in your daily routine; if you can do more, that is even better.

Regular exercise reduces the risk of breast cancer for both premenopausal and postmenopausal women. Regular physical activity, such as walking or cycling, is likely to reduce risk in numerous ways. It can enhance immunological function, which aids the body in fighting cancer-related infections. It can aid in maintaining healthy hormone levels (such as estrogen and progesterone) in the blood. And it can help women maintain a healthy weight. For colon cancer, the primary reason appears to be that exercise helps regulate insulin levels, which can keep specific hormones and growth factors that promote cancer in colon tissue under check.

Growing data suggest that beginning regular exercise early in life reduces the risk of developing breast cancer in adults. The period between the beginning of a girl's period and the birth of her first kid is crucial for the growth and development of her breasts. During this time, breast tissue appears to be more vulnerable to unfavorable risk factors, which presents an important chance to reduce the risk of adult breast cancer through a balanced diet, physical activity, and weight maintenance.

Protect Yourself Against the Sun: Melanoma, one of the deadliest forms of skin cancer, is one of the most prevalent types of cancer. As the incidence of melanoma rises consistently from year to year in both the United States and internationally, sun protection is a crucial public health message. Skin cancer is among the most preventable forms of cancer. Try the following:

- **Avoid noon sun.** Avoid the sun between 10 a.m. and 4 p.m., when its rays are at their maximum.

- **Remain under the shade.** When outdoors, you should spend as much time as possible in the shade. Sunglasses and a wide-brimmed hat are also beneficial.

- **Protect vulnerable skin areas.** Wear loose-fitting, tightly woven clothing that covers as much skin as possible. Choose vibrant or dark hues, which reflect more UV rays than pastels or white cotton.

- **Do not skimp on sunscreen.** Even on cloudy days, use a broad-spectrum sunscreen with an SPF of at least 30.

Apply sunscreen liberally and reapply it every two hours, or more frequently if swimming or perspiring.

- **Avoid tanning beds and sunlamps.** Also of concern is the use of tanning beds, particularly among adolescents and young adults. The International Association for Research on Cancer classifies indoor tanning as carcinogenic to humans, and the growth in indoor tanning closely parallels the increase in melanoma prevalence. The use of tanning beds raised the risk of melanoma by around 20 percent, according to a meta-analysis of the data of various research. If use began before the age of 35, the risk increased by 90 percent. These are equally destructive as natural sunlight.

Avoid Risky Behaviours: Avoiding dangerous activities that can result in infections, which may raise the risk of cancer, is another excellent cancer preventive strategy. For example:

- **Practice safe sex**. Limit the number of sexual partners you have and always use a condom. The greater the number of sexual partners you have in your lifetime, the higher your risk of contracting a sexually transmitted infection, such as HIV or HPV. People with HIV or AIDS are more likely to develop cancers of the anus, liver, and lungs. HPV is most commonly connected with cervical cancer, but it may also increase the risk of cancers of the anus, penis, throat, vulva, and vagina.

- Sharing needles with intravenous drug users can result in HIV, hepatitis B, and hepatitis C, which can raise the risk of liver cancer. If you have concerns about drug abuse or addiction, you should seek professional assistance.

If at all, consume alcohol in moderation: Alcohol has multiple effects on health. While studies have shown that even moderate alcohol use can increase the risk of two major malignancies (breast and colon), there is also strong evidence that moderate alcohol consumption can dramatically reduce the risk of cardiovascular disease in older persons. The trick is to balance these risks and advantages. Although the benefits of moderate alcohol consumption in older persons are well-established, non-drinkers should not be urged to start drinking due to the cancer risk and potential for alcohol dependence. The majority of adults who drink moderately do not need to stop. All heavy drinkers, however, should be encouraged to reduce their consumption to reasonable levels or abstain entirely. Growing data suggest that drinking during adolescence and young adulthood has a significant impact on breast cancer risk in later life. Youth should never consume alcohol. Young adult women should ideally abstain from alcohol, but if they do drink, they should limit their intake to moderate or lower levels and avoid binge drinking.

Alcohol likely increases the risk of breast cancer and colon cancer by decreasing folate levels in the body, although there are other probable explanations. Several studies have demonstrated that folic acid protects against cancer. Therefore, the lower levels generated by alcohol may increase the danger.

Evidence suggests that taking a folate supplement (such as a multivitamin) may reduce some of the cancer risks associated with alcohol consumption.

Avoid Contracting Infections: Infections play a significant influence in the development of various malignancies, although being largely unknown to the public. Infections are associated with approximately 23 percent of all malignancies in lower-income nations, 7 percent in higher-income countries, and 4 percent in North America.

Certain infections can directly or indirectly result in the development of cancer-causing mutations. This may occur because of the chronic inflammation caused by certain illnesses or because an infectious agent (such as a virus) modifies the behavior of infected cells. Infections that impair the immune system (such as HIV) raise the risk of cancer by reducing the body's ability to protect against cancer-causing infections.

The health burden of infection-associated malignancies is not shared equally by everybody. The poor living conditions and inadequate health care encountered by a significant portion of the global population enhance the chance of cancer caused by chronic infections. At least eleven infectious agents are known to raise the risk of cancer, and a number of them are extremely prevalent. However, in most cases, only a small percentage of people infected go on to acquire cancer since it needs a unique combination of conditions in addition to the infection to transform normal cells into malignant ones.

Nonetheless, these infectious pathogens have a large global impact on cancer. Human papillomavirus (HPV), hepatitis B and C viruses, and Helicobacter pylori are of particular importance. HPV is a sexually transmitted virus that has been associated with a number of malignancies, the most significant of which is cervical cancer. According to estimates, nearly all cervical malignancies are caused by HPV infection. Hepatitis B and C infect the liver and are responsible for the vast majority of cases of liver cancer. The stomach-infecting bacteria Helicobacter pylori is estimated to be responsible for up to 75 percent of all stomach cancers, the fourth most prevalent malignancy worldwide.

The prospect of cancer prevention is a bright spot when considering the scope of malignancies caused by infections. Girls and boys vaccinated against HPV can prevent cervical cancer as well as penile, anal, and throat cancers. The increasingly used hepatitis B vaccine helps prevent liver cancer. The treatment of Helicobacter pylori reduces the incidence of stomach cancer. And enhanced Hepatitis C screening and treatment may reduce liver cancer risk.

Vaccinate yourself: Cancer prevention involves protection against some viral diseases. Consult your physician for vaccination against:

- **Hepatitis B.** Hepatitis B can heighten the likelihood of getting liver cancer. The hepatitis B vaccine is recommended for certain high-risk adults, including those who are sexually active but not in a mutually monogamous relationship, those with sexually transmitted infections, those who use intravenous drugs, men who have sex with men, and health care or public safety personnel who may be exposed to infected blood or body fluids.

- **Human papillomavirus (HPV).** HPV is a sexually transmitted virus that can cause cervical and other genital cancers, as well as head-and-neck squamous cell carcinomas. The HPV vaccine is recommended for 11- and 12-year-old girls and boys. The U.S. Food and Drug Administration has officially authorized Gardasil 9 for use in males and females aged 9 to 45.

Total or Full Body Check-Up: A full body check-up is a comprehensive health examination or diagnostic scan of your entire body, including your heart, kidney, liver, and lungs, to evaluate your current health state and screen you for any obvious warning signals or abnormalities within your body. If there are symptoms of fatal diseases such as cardiovascular diseases, respiratory diseases, cancer, diabetes, high blood pressure, digestive diseases, etc., a health examination can sound the alarm. At least once a year, everyone should have a full-body examination to determine their health and identify any abnormalities or disorders. It can also alert you to unhealthy habits and encourage you to adopt a healthy lifestyle.

Why a Total Body Exam is Necessary:

- Individuals over the age of 35 should undergo a regular, comprehensive health examination.

- A full body examination is of the utmost importance, particularly in the case of severe and fatal conditions such as cancer, where an early diagnosis could help us prevent or control the disease and prolong the patient's life.

- A comprehensive bodily examination should take precedence in cases of Pre-existing disease history; Family medical history; Anyone with an unhealthy and stressful lifestyle must get a thorough physical examination.

- The average human immune system is challenged by high levels of pollution and novel methods of food contamination and adulteration, hence; a preventative health exam proved to be the optimal approach.

A comprehensive health examination could include a number of tests and skilled medical advice, inclusively; gynecology consultations (exclusively for females). In a nutshell, to enjoy a happy, healthy and carefree life, you must have regular health examinations. Remember the adage, **"Prevention is better than cure"**

CHAPTER 4

OTHER HELPFUL TIPS – Food and Cancer, Detoxification and Cancer; Stress Reduction, Sleep and Cancer

FOOD AND CANCER

No single item can prevent cancer, but consuming the appropriate balance of foods may help. The foods we consume can influence our susceptibility to acquiring certain types of cancer. High-calorie, high-fat diets can cause obesity and are believed to raise the risk of certain malignancies. Eating a wide variety of foods from each food group in the prescribed amounts helps maintain a balanced and fascinating diet and provides the body with a variety of nutrients. Eating a variety of foods boosts health and reduces the risk of developing some diseases. Below are some lists of foods that may reduce the risk of cancer.

Color in Cancer Prevention: The more vibrant the color of fruits and vegetables, the more cancer-fighting elements they contain. These meals can also reduce your risk by assisting you in achieving and maintaining a healthy body weight. Multiple cancers, including colon, oesophageal, and kidney tumors, are associated with carrying additional weight. Consume a variety of veggies, particularly those that are dark green, red, and orange.

The Cancer-Fighting Breakfast: Folate is an essential B vitamin that may help prevent colon, rectum, and breast cancers. On the breakfast table, it can be found in plenty. Fortified morning cereals and items made with whole wheat are excellent sources of folate. Also, orange juice, melons, strawberries; asparagus, and eggs are more foods that are rich in folate. Beans, sunflower seeds, and leafy green vegetables such as spinach and romaine lettuce also contain vitamin K. The best source of folate is not a pill, but a diet rich in fruits, vegetables, and grain products. Pregnant or potentially pregnant women should take a folic acid supplement to avoid certain birth abnormalities.

Processed Meat Consumption: Reducing your consumption of processed meats such as bologna, ham, and hot dogs will reduce your risk of colorectal and stomach cancers. Additionally, consuming smoked or salted meats increases your exposure to substances that have the potential to cause cancer.

Tomatoes Against Cancer: It is unclear if the pigment lycopene, which gives tomatoes their red color, or something else is responsible. Nonetheless, a number of studies have connected the consumption of tomatoes to a decreased risk of cancer, particularly prostate cancer. Studies also indicate that processed tomato products, such as juice, sauce, and paste, have anti-cancer properties.

Green Tea: Even if the research is inconclusive, tea, especially green tea, may be a potent cancer fighter, especially if it contains polyphenols.

Green tea has slowed or prevented the growth of cancer in colon, liver, breast, and prostate cells in laboratory experiments. It showed a comparable impact on lung tissue and skin. In certain long-term studies, tea consumption was connected with a reduced incidence of bladder, stomach, and pancreatic cancer.

Grapes And Cancer: Grapes and grape juice contain resveratrol, particularly purple and red grapes. Resveratrol possesses powerful anti-inflammatory and antioxidant effects. In laboratory experiments, it has been shown to prevent cell damage that can initiate the cancer process. There is insufficient evidence to conclude that consuming grapes, grape juice, or wine (or taking dietary supplements) can prevent or treat cancer, but the health benefits of taking them once in a while cannot be over-emphasized.

Water and Other Fluids Can Protect: In addition to quenching your thirst, water may also protect you from bladder cancer. Water dilutes quantities of probable cancer-causing chemicals in the bladder, reducing the risk. Additionally, drinking more fluids increases the frequency of urination which in turn flushes the body systems of toxins. This reduces the amount of time these drugs are exposed to the bladder lining.

The Cabbage Family and Cancer: Broccoli, cauliflower, cabbage, Brussels sprouts, bok choy, and kale are cruciferous vegetables. These members of the cabbage family make a great stir-fry and can enliven a salad tremendously.

Moreover, these vegetables may help your body defend itself against malignancies such as colon, breast, lung, and cervix.

Dark green leafy vegetables, including mustard greens, lettuce, kale, chicory, spinach, and chard, are rich in fiber, folate, and carotenoids. These nutrients may help prevent oral, laryngeal, pancreatic, lung, skin, and stomach cancer.

Cooking Method Is Crucial: The way in which meat is prepared affects the cancer risk it poses. When frying, grilling, or broiling meats at extremely high temperatures, cancer-causing compounds are produced. Other cooking techniques, such as braising, stewing, and steaming, appear to release less of these compounds. And when you stew the meat, be sure to include an abundance of nutritious vegetables.

Do not Consume Sugar: Sugar may not directly cause cancer; however, it may displace other cancer-preventing meals high in nutrients. It also raises calorie counts, which adds to obesity and overweight. Additionally, obesity poses a cancer risk. Fruit provides a healthy alternative to sugary foods.

Avoid Over Dependence on Supplements: Vitamins may aid in cancer prevention, however; this is when they are obtained organically through food. Both the American Cancer Society and the American Institute for Cancer Research highlight that obtaining cancer-fighting elements, vitamins, and minerals from fresh foods such as nuts, fruits, and green leafy vegetables is much superior to supplementation. A healthy diet is optimal.

DETOXIFICATION AND CANCER

Our bodies are continuously exposed to toxins, ranging from ambient pollutants to chemical toxins produced by the body during normal function. If the body is unable to detoxify itself adequately, the accumulation of toxins frequently causes cellular damage and inflammation, which increases the chance of developing major chronic diseases, such as cancer.

Detoxification is the process of removing and purifying the body of harmful substances. A detoxification program aims to prevent and reverse cellular damage, which, if left unchecked, can pose major health hazards. Effective detoxification results in improved overall health, vitality, energy, and well-being. Regular detoxification is essential for cellular renewal and longevity.

The human body contains the capacity to cleanse itself. In actuality, the body contains several waste removal mechanisms. Skin, liver, lungs, large intestine, and kidneys are the primary organs that make up the waste elimination system. Blood, intestines, and lymph play crucial functions in maintaining the equilibrium between health and illness. For a variety of reasons, natural detoxification may not adequately clear toxins from the body, hence the need for additional detoxification measures.

A number of detoxification regimens are available within an integrated health care model. The following are a few techniques for eliminating toxins from your body in the comfort of your own home:

- Exercise and movement
- Body-mind equilibrium (yoga, meditation, breathing, prayer)
- Early morning water therapy (room temperature or warm water)
- Fasting, Juicing, Supplements (naturally derived primarily from fresh fruits and vegetables)
- Detox Massages, Body Scrubs, and numerous others.

Every day, our system automatically detoxifies by eliminating accumulated waste. If the body's ability to eliminate toxic waste is less than the toxic overload, cells begin to malfunction due to free radicals, an inflammatory by-product, and the illness process begins. Eliminating excessive toxins and the health risks they pose requires detoxification. On the premise that the build-up of toxins significantly contributes to cellular damage and disease formation, the elimination of toxins has the potential to prevent and potentially reverse this grave health danger.

STRESS REDUCTION, SLEEP, AND CANCER

Stress is universal, but chronic stress is distinct. Long-lasting emotional strain is the cause of chronic stress. This can boost the release of stress hormones, resulting in mental and physical issues. Many individuals diagnosed with cancer have an increase in stress, which can easily become chronic. Recent research indicates that persistent stress may potentially accelerate the spread of cancer. The spreading of cancer throughout the body can be accelerated by stress, particularly ovarian, breast, and colorectal cancers. When the body experiences stress, neurotransmitters such as norepinephrine are released, which promote the growth of cancer cells. This stimulation can help cancer cells elude death, proliferate, and adapt to new settings, allowing them to thrive in new locations. Chronic stress severely compromises the immune system, which is already compromised by cancer treatment. A compromised immune system promotes disease and infection vulnerability.

Additionally, chronic stress can cause sadness and anxiety. A negative view of life can be detrimental to the body and mind. People with anxiety and depression may engage in harmful stress management strategies. Others cope with stress by drinking or smoking, and some overeat. Depression can produce weariness, which frequently leads to a lack of physical activity. All of these practices can lead to health problems that can cause cancer.

Stress can be managed healthily, but it increases the likelihood of adopting unhealthy behaviors.

A Simple Introductory Relaxation Technique:

- Sit or recline and make yourself comfortable. Let your arms rest at your sides, and do not cross your legs. (Initially, it is beneficial to eliminate as many distractions as possible; a dark, silent area is helpful. With practice, letting go becomes increasingly simple, even under less-than-ideal circumstances.) Stretch and wiggle your muscles until you feel more at ease, then, close your eyes lightly.

- Take a steady, deep breath through your nose, allowing your lungs and stomach to fill with air. When your lungs are full, hold your breath for a brief moment, and then slowly exhale, feeling yourself let go all over. When you feel the air leaving your lungs, do not rush to inhale; instead, take a steady, smooth, deep breath, feel yourself filling up, hold it for a second, and then exhale slowly and thoroughly to further relax. Exhale for a longer duration than your intake, and truly let go. Get immersed and absorbed in simply listening to your breaths and letting go of your body. Perform this for a few more breaths, and then breathe normally, without attempting to inhale particularly deeply. Ensure that you are breathing deeply rather than shallowly (just from the chest).

- Allow your focus to settle on your toes. Slowly and softly contract the toe muscles.

Feel the tightness, then let the toes relax and see the difference. Observe the sensations you feel in your toes as you relax them.

- Repeat this pattern of tensing and relaxing each major muscle group as you ascend the body: calves, thighs, hips, abdomen, back, shoulders, arms, neck, jaws, eyes, forehead, and scalp. As you grew engrossed in your breathing, lose yourself in the feelings you make by directly relaxing all of your muscles.

- After working on each muscle group individually, stretch your arms and legs and contract all of your muscles simultaneously (or as many as you can). Then, let your body relax. Take several calm, deep breaths. If you feel any lingering tension in any part of your body, repeat the tense-and-relax cycle in that place to see if you can loosen it.

- Lastly, prior to opening your eyes, take a little voyage throughout your body, noting how deeply relaxed you feel. Become accustomed to the sensation. When you are ready, take another deep breath and open your eyes slowly.

Slow, deep breathing and general muscular relaxation are two of the simplest and most direct techniques for calming down. Most of us breathe between sixteen and twenty times per minute; by breathing slowly and deeply, we can lower this amount in half or more.

Combined with muscular relaxation, the final impact is to slow the heart rate, reduce blood pressure, relax the muscles, and increase blood flow to the hands and feet; in other words, to generate the reverse of the stressful fight-or-flight response. This relaxing method can be approached in numerous ways. A useful technique is to silently repeat a sound, word, or phrase in time with your breathing, such as "I am..." (as you inhale) "... calm" (as you breathe out).

Imagine yourself in a quiet, enjoyable situation, such as a warm beach, a lush green meadow, a refreshing mountain lake, or floating on a fluffy white cloud. The trick is to maintain simplicity and enjoyment. If the procedure is not pleasurable, it is likely to be ineffective and will not be completed. Making it a chore will only serve to heighten your anxiety. Along with diet, sleep, and exercise, stress reduction should be seen as a crucial factor in preserving health and preventing disease.

Many of us have learned that a diet rich in fresh vegetables, fruits, and whole grains, daily exercise, and sun protection can dramatically reduce our risk of developing cancer. On the list of strategies to prevent cancer, quitting smoking and consuming less alcohol rank high. But how frequently do we recognize that sufficient sleep is required to maintain a healthy immune system and prevent the development of cancer? Do we actively handle stress in our daily lives so that its negative effects on our bodies and minds do not harm us?

In a society in which women and men are encouraged to "lean in," run faster, and aim higher, it is essential to recognize the importance of excellent sleep and stress reduction. What relevance does this have with cancer? Simply said, our bodies and minds are intimately intertwined, and anything that impacts our mental state will invariably alter how our bodies work. For this reason, good sleep and stress reduction play a vital role in cancer prevention. A renowned cancer researcher told me, "Every day we battle cancer cells." To win this battle, we must strengthen and maintain our immune systems.

Our bodies require sufficient sleep to rejuvenate and safeguard the state of our immune systems and minds, which is not surprising. Insufficient sleep causes a rise in cortisol and hunger hormones, which in turn causes an increase in insulin. Diverse hormones, including leptin, melatonin, growth hormone, testosterone, and serotonin, decrease, resulting in weight increase. When we stay up beyond midnight, our hormones become unbalanced, causing us to eat more frequently. 10 p.m. is regarded to be the ideal hour to begin sleeping at night. How can we optimize our nightly sleep? Before night, turn off cell phones, computers, and televisions, as well as any other distracting gadgets, to create a tranquil and pleasant environment. The conclusion of exercise, eating, and drinking should occur several hours before bedtime. Avoid drinking caffeinated beverages in the evening if possible.

As soon as we arise, we should let natural light into our homes. Melatonin, a critical hormone involved in sleeping and waking, should be at its lowest level in the early morning. Persistent darkness will keep your body's melatonin levels up, causing you to feel sleepy and difficult to completely awaken. As the day begins, we are confronted with natural stressors related to our family, workplace, bosses, friends, and others. Although we cannot avoid stress entirely in our daily lives, we can learn how to manage it effectively. Possessing a supportive network of family and friends and maintaining a happy view of life can also assist enhance the immune system. There are numerous ways to lower cancer risk every day, although a direct connection between stress and cancer development has not been fully demonstrated. Nonetheless, it makes sense to maintain and support a strong immune system that can combat numerous diseases.

CONCLUSION

Cancer is not a singular illness; rather, it is accompanied by a myriad of additional health problems. Cancer comes in a wide variety of forms and sub-forms; while certain cancers are more dangerous than others, there are a number of factors that can contribute to the development of unique cancer characteristics. In light of the result contained in your pathology report, your oncologist will be able to provide you with a clearer comprehension of the normal behavior of a particular type of cancer.

Breast cancer is the second most frequent type of cancer in the United States, after nonmelanoma skin cancer. On the other hand, lung cancer is the most common type of cancer to result in mortality. The treatments are consistently getting better. Chemotherapy, radiation therapy, and surgery are some examples of contemporary treatment modalities. Some individuals find that more recent treatment alternatives, such as stem cell transplantation and precision medicine, are beneficial to their health. As a result of advances in cancer screening, therapy, and prevention, survival rates are going up for a variety of cancers. Cancer is a disease that can be successfully treated for a large number of patients, the survival rate after therapy for cancer is higher than it has ever been previously. *'Having given birth to seven children, my mother was diagnosed with breast cancer and was treated through surgery, years later, she had another child and went through the process of breastfeeding, till today; she is still alive and in good health'.* Even though cancer may be fatal, effective treatment and prevention is still hundred percent possible.